What Lou Can Do

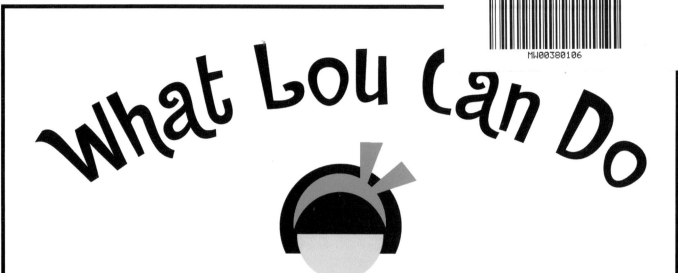

How nutrition, exercise and motivation can put
you on the good path to healthy living.

Story by Christine Audler

Illustrations by Mark Andresen

There once was a girl named Lou,
who didn't know what to do.
She ate everything yummy.
She grew a big tummy.
Then couldn't fit into her shoes.

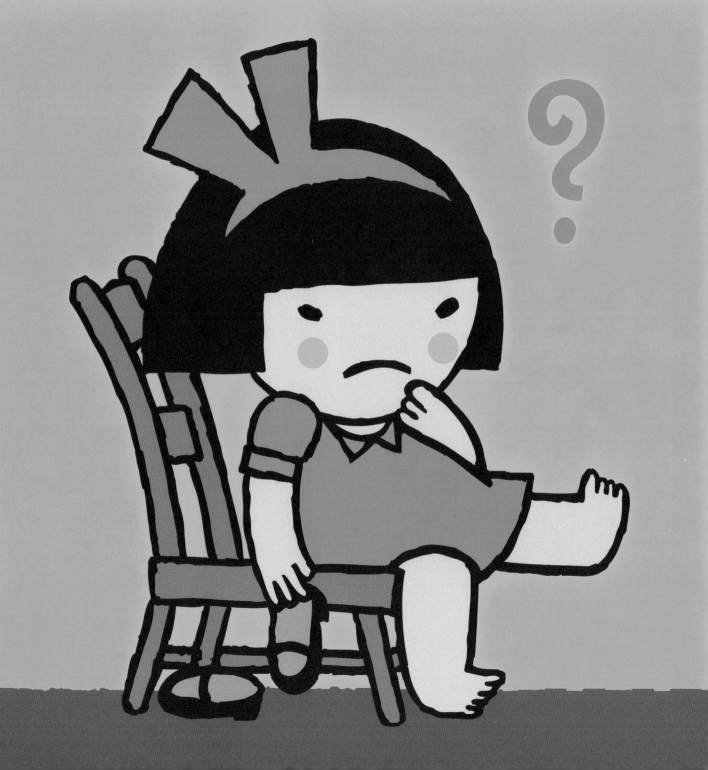

When served salad and peas,
Lou just loved her Chee Zees.
When offered a piece of fruit,
she gave her Mom the boot!!!

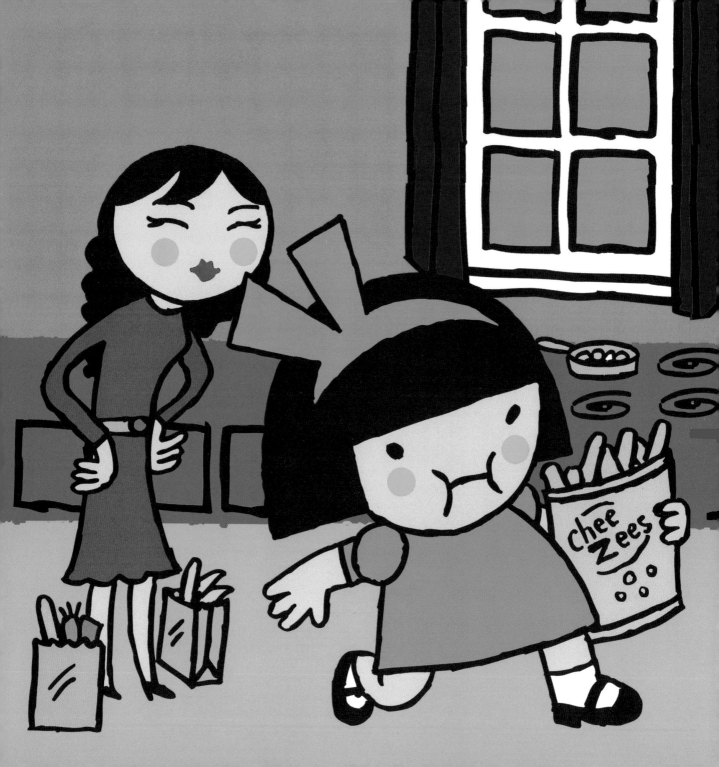

She didn't get lean,
she was glued to
the screen.

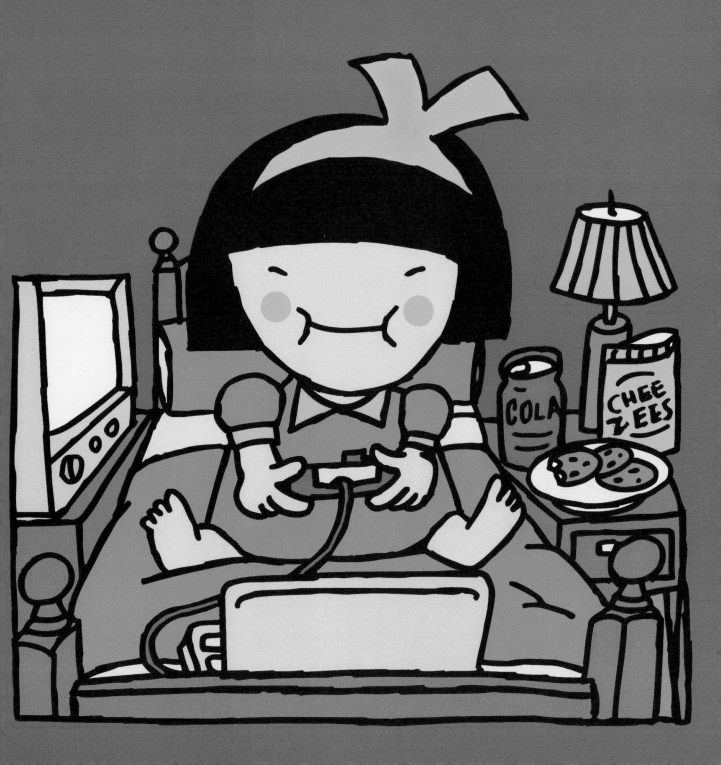

When she went to school,
she learned a golden rule:
There really is a simple way:
just eat right and lots of play!!!

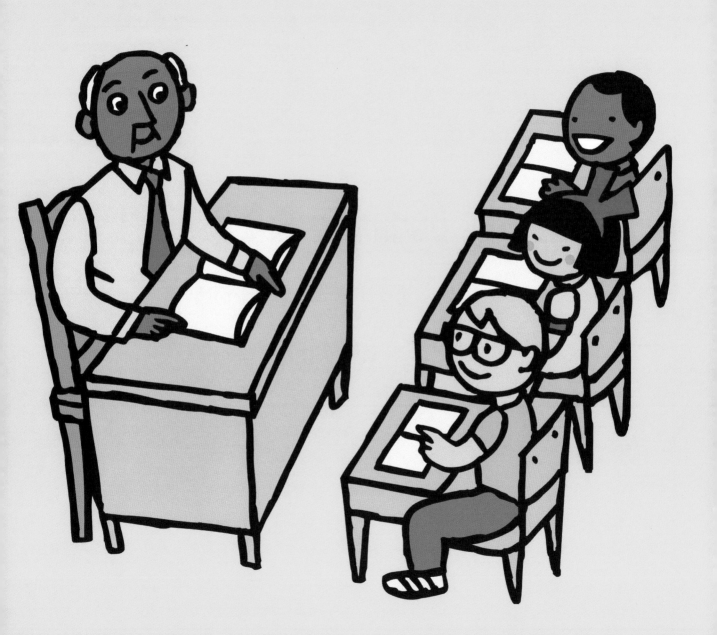

So, she began to eat healthy,
and started to feel
real wealthy!!!

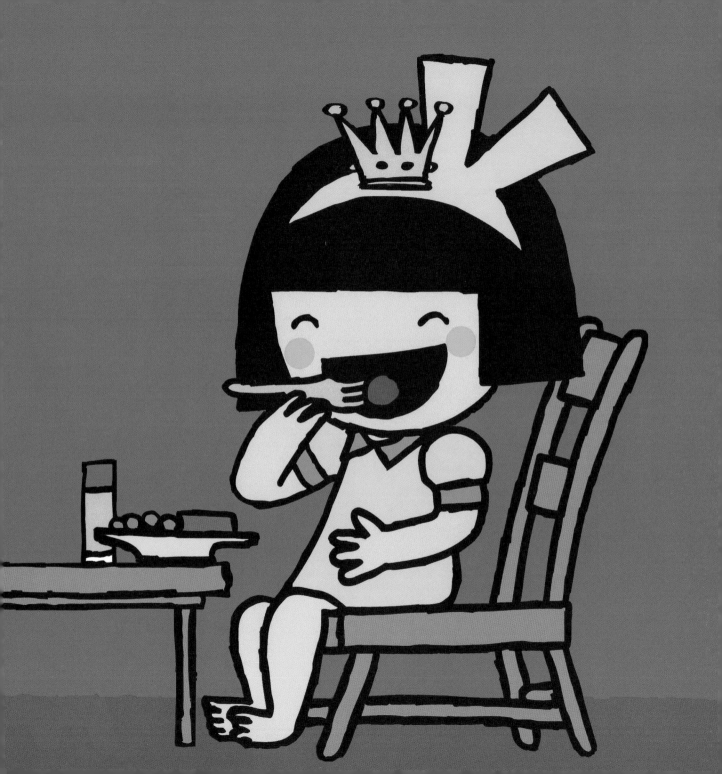

Lou began to play
and sweat all the pounds
away.

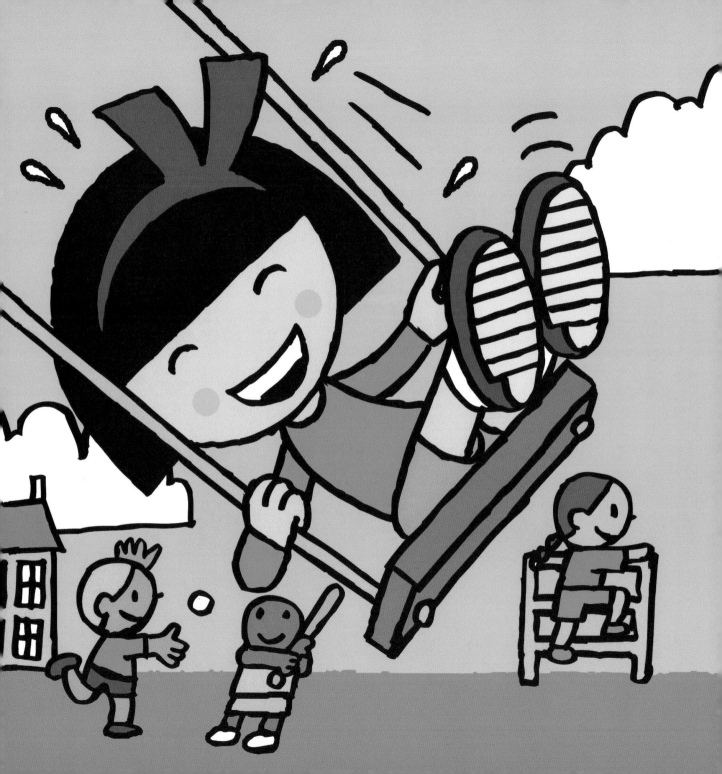

Now fit from head to toe,
Lou wants you to know:
You can fit inside your shoes,
if you just believe
in what you can do.

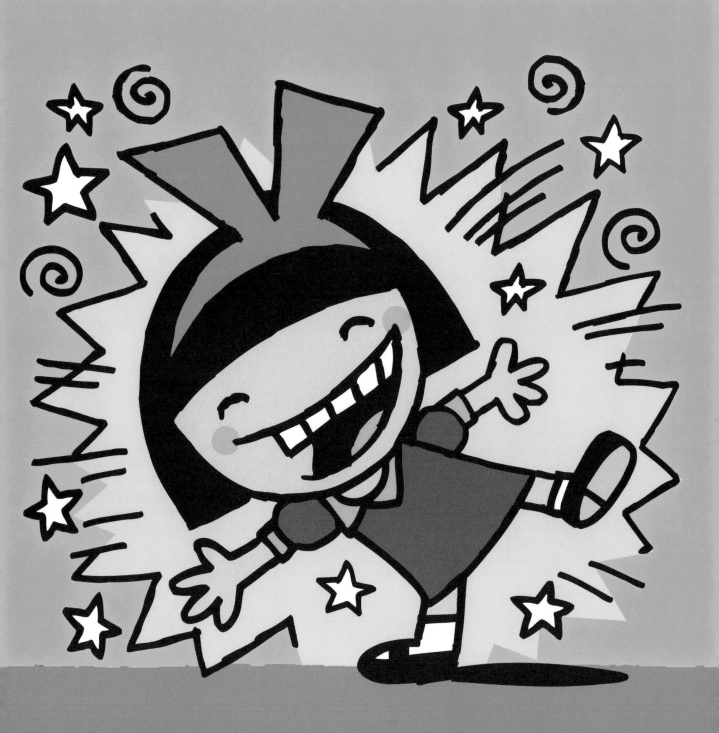

With healthy eating
and playing outside,
Lou discovered
who was truly INSIDE.

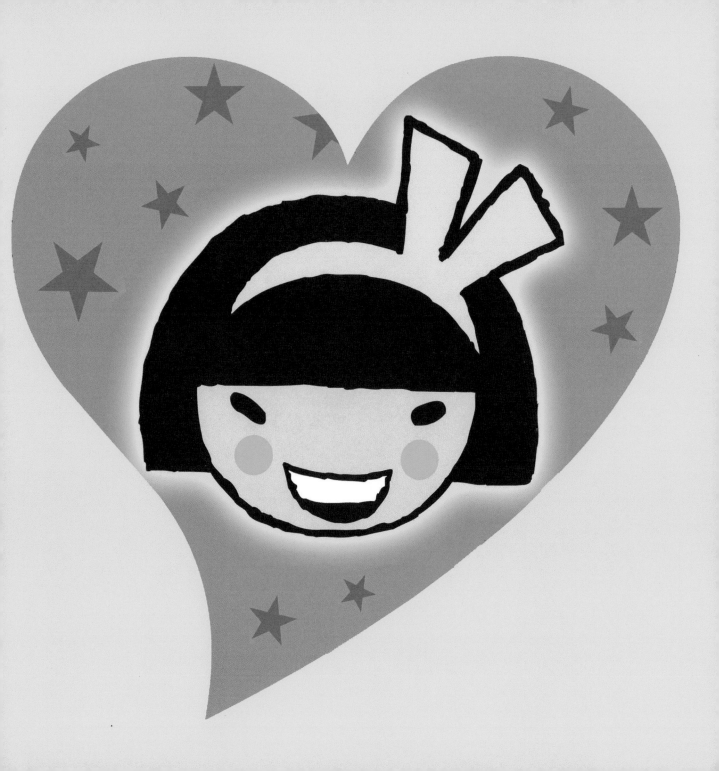

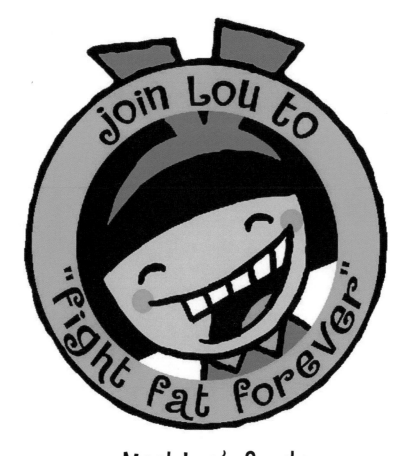

Meet Lou's family

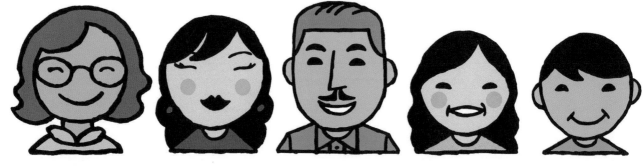

| Abuela | Mom | Dad | Lucy | Luke |

Help pick out today's activities for Lou by circling what she should do.

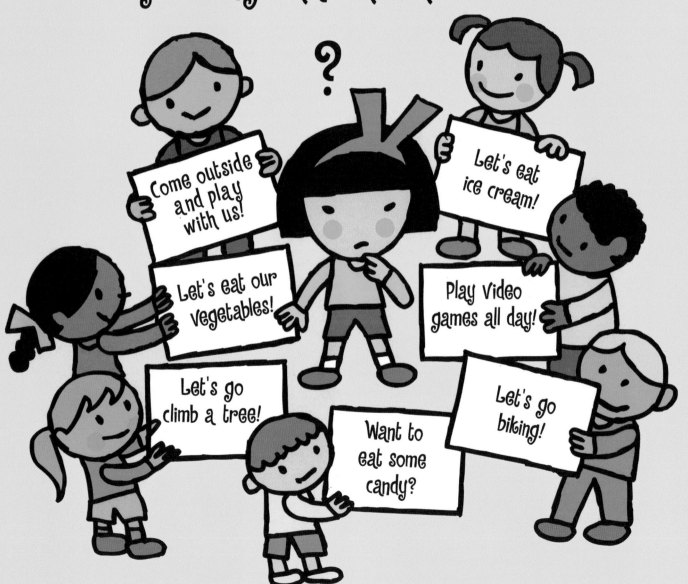

Circle 5 of your favorite foods and then see if they're healthy choices

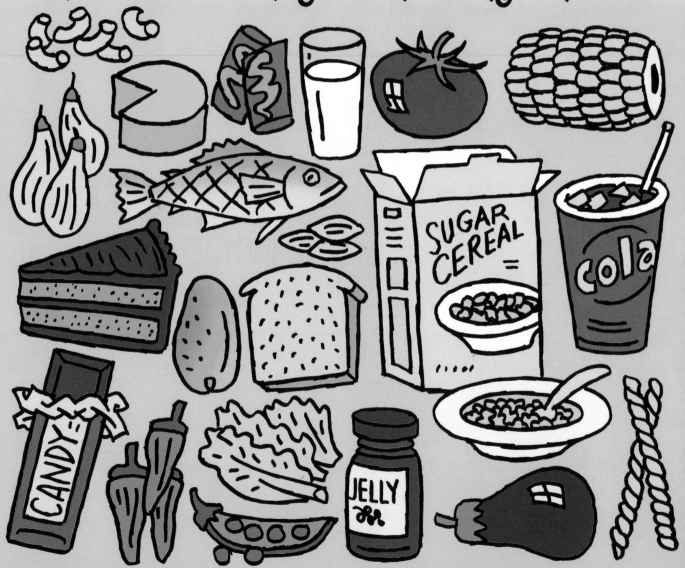

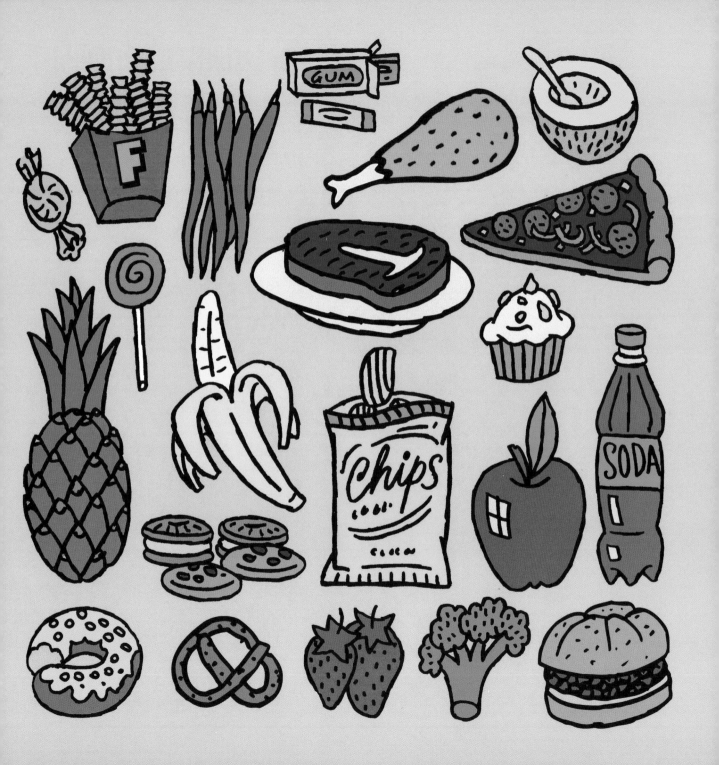

Wrong junk food choices

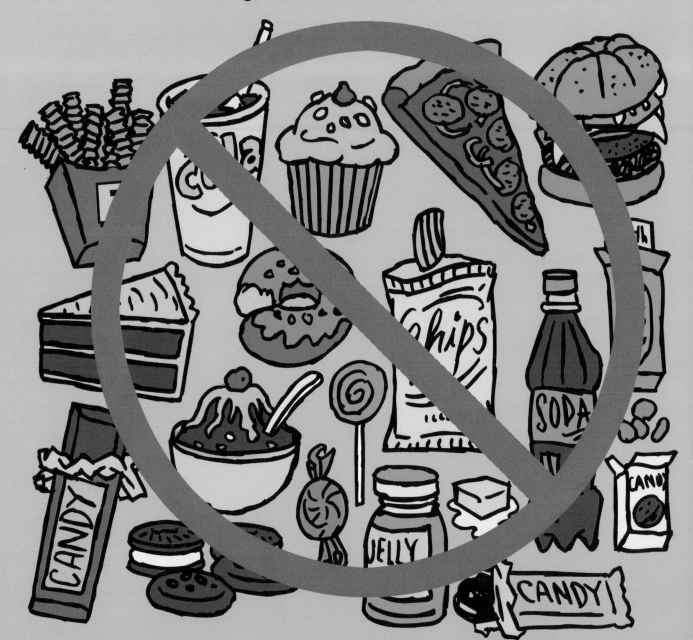